Pulsed Electromagnetic Field Therapy (PEMF)

Delving Into The Diverse Health Benefits Of PEMF Therapy.

TABLE OF CONTENT

INTRODUCTION

Overview of Pulsed Electromagnetic Field Therapy (PEMF)

At the nexus of science and medicine, pulsed electromagnetic field therapy, or PEMF, offers a cutting-edge method of improving health and well-being. Fundamentally, pulsed electromagnetic fields (PEMF) are used to maximize the body's inherent healing processes by stimulating and optimizing pulsating waves of energy. This therapeutic approach is becoming more and more well-known and accepted in complementary and mainstream medicine, offering a non-invasive, drug-free treatment option for a range of illnesses.

PEMF works on the premise that charged particles within the body, especially at the cellular level, are influenced by electromagnetic fields. In essence, the human body is a complex network of cells that communicate with one another via electrical signals. PEMF aims to modify these cellular signals by applying particular electromagnetic field intensities and frequencies, therefore fostering equilibrium and homeostasis.

PEMF has the potential to be used in many different health applications. Healthcare experts and anyone looking for complementary and alternative approaches to health and well-being have become interested in PEMF therapy due to its adaptability in treating chronic pain, stimulating tissue regeneration, enhancing sleep quality, and lowering stress levels.

This section will examine the basic ideas behind PEMF therapy, including how electromagnetic fields interact with the body, the physiological reactions they cause, and the wide spectrum of health advantages it offers. We must establish a strong basis for comprehending the complex dance between electromagnetic energy and the complex biology of the human body before we set out on this adventure.

Historical Evolution and Milestones

It is crucial to understand the historical development and turning points of PEMF therapy to completely comprehend its relevance. The idea of harnessing electromagnetic radiation for healing is not new; in fact, it has origins in ancient civilizations. Historical accounts indicate that societies like the Greeks and Egyptians of antiquity were aware of the therapeutic benefits of magnets. Nonetheless, the methodical investigation and advancement of PEMF therapy occurred during the past century.

Famous physicist Nikola Tesla's groundbreaking work in the early 20th century involved experimenting with electromagnetic fields, which set the foundation for modern PEMF technology. Future scientists and medical professionals will be able to investigate the curative potential of electromagnetic fields in a more focused and regulated way thanks to Tesla's innovative concepts and experiments.

Electromagnetic field science research gained momentum in the second half of the 20th century. Advances in technology have made it possible for scientists to investigate the molecular and cellular consequences of electromagnetic stimulation in more detail. A turning point was reached in the 1970s and 1980s when research showing the beneficial effects of PEMF on a range of biological processes was published.

The development of PEMF devices and their use followed technological advancements. PEMF technology has evolved through time through constant invention and improvement, from early experimental setups to the creation of portable and user-friendly devices. These days, PEMF devices are available in a variety of shapes and sizes, from specialized applicators to mats and pads, giving people a wide range of ways to incorporate this therapy into their daily routines.

This historical investigation not only honors the trailblazers who established PEMF therapy but also illustrates the process from conception to widespread use. Comprehending this progression is essential to recognizing the scientific validity and advancements that support the current use of PEMF in healthcare.

Purpose and Scope of the Book

Before we get into this in-depth examination of pulsed electromagnetic field therapy, let me make clear what this book is about and what its parameters are. The principal aim of this study is to provide readers with a comprehensive comprehension of PEMF, enabling them to make well-informed judgments on the integration of this therapy into their lives.

The following goals are pursued by the book:

- **Education and Awareness**

To give readers a comprehensive understanding of the fundamental ideas behind PEMF therapy, including an explanation of how electromagnetic fields interact with the body and the science underlying it. By raising awareness, readers are more equipped to make decisions about their health and consider PEMF as an adjunct to traditional therapies.

- **Practical Guidance**

Provide helpful advice on how to choose and use PEMF devices. This involves taking into account one's health objectives, unique medical problems, and an assessment of technical requirements. The book seeks to simplify the process of incorporating PEMF therapy into a daily routine by offering concise and useful information.

- **Safety and Precautions**

Talk about the safety issues and measures related to PEMF therapy. Even though PEMF is usually regarded as safe, several recommendations and contraindications need to be followed. The knowledge in this book will enable readers to use PEMF devices properly, reducing risks and optimizing benefits.

- **Exploration of Case Studies**

Examine real-world case studies and success tales to provide readers with an understanding of how PEMF therapy has helped people. These stories offer concrete instances of the many uses and results connected to PEMF, demonstrating its capacity to have a favorable effect on a range of medical diseases.

- **Future Trends and Developments**

Give an overview of the prospects for PEMF therapy going forward by going over current studies, new uses, and possible technological developments. By keeping up to date with the always-changing PEMF scene, readers can put themselves in a position to profit from the latest advancements in this field.

CHAPTER 1: FOUNDATIONS OF PEMF THERAPY

Understanding Electromagnetic Fields

It is vital to first investigate the underlying nature of electromagnetic fields to acquire an understanding of the basis of Pulsed Electromagnetic Field (PEMF) therapy. The movement of charged particles is what causes electromagnetic fields, which are ubiquitous forces that surround us, to be formed. Both the operation of the natural world and the fabric of our cosmos are dependent upon these fields, which play an essential part in both of these aspects.

Natural vs. Artificial EMFs

Electromagnetic Fields That Are Produced Naturally The Earth itself produces an electromagnetic field that is both complex and dynamic. The movement of molten iron within the outer core of the Earth is the cause of the magnetic field that surrounds the planet, which is also commonly referred to as the geomagnetic field. Everything from the migration habits of animals to the functioning of the human brain is influenced by this natural field.

Unlike natural electromagnetic fields, artificial electromagnetic fields are produced by human-made sources such as power lines, electrical appliances, and wireless communication devices. These fields are characterized by their ability to generate electromagnetic fields. These artificial fields constitute an essential component of contemporary living; yet, there have been concerns expressed about the potential adverse effects on health, which has led to the investigation of therapeutic uses such as pulsed electromagnetic fields (PEMF).

Basic Principles of Electromagnetism

Fundamentally, a set of rules that define the connection between electric charges and magnetic fields control electromagnetism. Important ideas consist of:

The relationship between the flow of electric current and the magnetic fields it produces is known as Ampere's Law. It proves that a conductor carrying current creates a magnetic field surrounding it.

Faraday's Law: This law explains how electromagnetic induction occurs. Conductors experience electric currents when their magnetic fields change. Many electrical gadgets operate on this fundamental idea.

James Clerk Maxwell developed the equations known as Maxwell's Equations, which combine the concepts of electricity and magnetism. They lay the groundwork for classical electromagnetism by describing the interactions and spatial propagation of electric and magnetic fields.

THE SCIENCE BEHIND PEMF

How PEMF Influences Cellular Function

The key component of PEMF therapy is its cellular-level interaction with the organism. The fundamental units of life, cells, communicate using electrical signals. Several physiological reactions take place in response to PEMF, impacting cellular function and enhancing general well-being.

Cellular Resonance: The body's various cell types each have a resonance frequency at which they function best. The frequencies that PEMF devices generate are intended to resonate with certain cell types. This resonance can increase cellular activity and support homeostasis, which is a balanced condition.

Ion Exchange: PEMF can affect how ions pass through cell membranes. Maintaining the electrical potential of cells and ensuring appropriate cellular function depends on this ion exchange. This process can be aided by PEMF therapy, which helps to regulate cellular processes.

Enhanced Circulation: Blood flow and vascular function can be impacted by electromagnetic fields. PEMF supports cells' metabolic processes by enhancing microcirculation and inducing vasodilation, which improves oxygenation and nutrient delivery to cells.

Frequency, Intensity, and Waveforms

Frequency:

A key component of PEMF treatment is frequency, which is defined as the number of oscillations or cycles per unit of time. Different frequencies influence cellular processes in different ways, resulting in unique consequences on the body. Higher frequencies (100-1000 Hz) may be utilized to address certain health concerns, whereas lower frequencies (between 1-100 Hz) are frequently employed for general well-being and relaxation.

- Delta: (1-4 Hz): Linked to deep sleep and tissue repair.
- Theta (4–8 Hz): Associated with meditation and rest.

- Alpha (8–14 Hz): Promotes calmness and increased attention.
- Beta (14–30 Hz): Enhances cognitive function and attentiveness.

To get the most of the benefits of PEMF therapy, it is essential to have a thorough understanding of the therapeutic aims and to choose the most appropriate frequency.

Intensity:

The intensity of the magnetic field that is generated by a PEMF device is commonly measured in Gauss or Tesla. Intensity encompasses the strength of the magnetic field. One of the factors that determines the depth of penetration into tissues is the intensity of the field. Higher intensities may be appropriate for addressing disorders that are deeply rooted, however, lesser intensities are typically utilized for general well-being and applications that are more straightforward.

One thing that should be kept in mind is that the intensity level that is selected ought to be following the particular health objectives and conditions of the individual. Seeking the advice of a healthcare professional or an experienced practitioner can be of great assistance in determining the appropriate level of intensity for a certain circumstance.

Waveforms:

A PEMF signal's waveform shows how the oscillations are shaped. Waveforms that are frequently seen are sawtooth, square, and sinusoidal. Every waveform has distinct qualities that can affect how cells respond physiologically.

Sinusoidal: Said to be mild and well-tolerated, sinusoidal electromagnetic fields mimic natural electromagnetic fields.

Square: This is thought to have more direct impacts on cellular membranes and is characterized by quick polarity changes.

Sawtooth: Offers a balance between sensitivity and strength by combining features of square and sinusoidal waveforms.

Waveform selection is influenced by several variables, including individual sensitivity and the intended therapeutic result. Waveform parameter personalization improves PEMF therapy's applicability to a range of medical demands.

CHAPTER 2: HEALTH BENEFITS OF PEMF THERAPY

PEMF therapy, which stands for pulsed electromagnetic field therapy, has garnered a lot of attention due to the wide variety of health benefits it provides. It is a non-invasive and drug-free method of achieving well-being. Throughout this part, we will investigate the numerous benefits that PEMF therapy offers, providing light on how it positively affects various elements of health.

Pain Management and Relief

- **Chronic Pain Conditions**

The management and alleviation of disorders that cause chronic pain is one of the principal applications of pulsed electromagnetic field therapy (PEMF). A variety of conditions, including arthritis, fibromyalgia, and musculoskeletal problems, can be the cause of chronic pain, which is characterized by its persistent and incapacitating nature. It has been established that PEMF is effective in reducing pain by affecting the physiological systems that are at the root of the problem.

Cellular Resonance and Pain Perception:

Ion exchange and cellular resonance are both affected by PEMF's operation, which takes place at the cellular level. Pain-induced muscle contractions (PEMF) can affect pain perception by changing the electrical characteristics of cells, particularly nerve cells that are involved in pain signaling. The persistent pain that is linked with illnesses such as arthritis and neuropathy can be alleviated somewhat through the utilization of this mechanism.

Inflammation Reduction:

In many cases, the inflammatory processes are at the core of illnesses that cause chronic pain. There is evidence that pulsed electromagnetic fields (PEMF) have anti-inflammatory effects, which reduce the generation of chemicals that promote inflammation. This decrease in inflammation may provide relief from the discomfort associated with conditions including rheumatoid arthritis and inflammatory joint problems.

- **Inflammatory Pain**

Pulsed electromagnetic field (PEMF) therapy is beneficial in treating acute inflammatory pain in addition to chronic pain disorders. Pain and discomfort can be caused by injuries, surgical procedures, or inflammatory responses. There is a correlation between the ability of PEMF to control inflammatory pathways and a speedier resolution of acute pain, which in turn promotes a faster recovery.

- **Postoperative Pain Management:**

Some research has suggested that pulsed electromagnetic fields (PEMF) therapy may be useful for the management of postoperative pain. Through the reduction of inflammation, the promotion of tissue regeneration, and the modulation of pain perception, electrical muscle stimulation (PEMF) helps to make the healing process more comfortable.

Sports Injuries and Inflammation:

Frequently, athletes experience injuries that are accompanied by inflammation. Pulsed electromagnetic field (PEMF) therapy has been investigated as a supplemental method to hasten the healing process in sports-related injuries. This therapy provides a non-pharmacological alternative for the management of pain and the promotion of the recovery of injured tissues.

Accelerating Healing Processes

- **Bone and Tissue Regeneration**

Particularly remarkable in the context of bone and tissue repair are the regenerative characteristics that PEMF therapy possesses. The interaction of electromagnetic fields with the activities that occur within cells is an essential component in the process of triggering regeneration mechanisms.

Fracture Healing:

It has been demonstrated through research that PEMF therapy helps speed up the healing process of fractures. PEMF can hasten the production of new bone tissue by fostering the proliferation and differentiation of bone cells. This is especially helpful in situations where the fracture has not yet healed or has been delayed.

Osteoporosis Management:

A disorder that is characterized by weaker bones, osteoporosis, has been the subject of research into the potential of PEMF therapy as a treatment for the ailment. PEMF is a non-pharmacological method that can be used to promote bone health, particularly in persons who are prone to osteoporotic fractures. It does this by boosting bone density and remodeling.

- **Wound Healing**

The application of PEMF therapy extends to the healing of wounds, demonstrating its capacity to encourage the regenerative processes of the skin and the tissues that lie beneath it.

Enhanced Collagen Production:

Within the context of the process of wound healing, collagen is an essential component. It has been established that PEMF can stimulate the creation of collagen, which has the effect of contributing to the construction of a robust and resilient extracellular matrix at the site of the wound.

Improved Blood Flow:

When it comes to wound healing, the influence that PEMF has on blood circulation is favorable. By ensuring that the wound receives an adequate quantity of oxygen and nutrients, improved microcirculation helps to speed up the

healing process and reduce the likelihood of

problems occurring.

Enhancing Cellular Function

▪ ATP Production

ATP, which stands for adenosine triphosphate, is the energy currency that cells use. There is evidence that pulsed electromagnetic fields (PEMF) therapy can affect the generation of ATP, which has far-reaching ramifications for the function of cells and overall health.

Mitochondrial Stimulation:

The production of ATP is mostly dependent on mitochondria, which are known as the "powerhouses" of cells. PEMF therapy has been shown to improve mitochondrial function, which in turn leads to an increase in the synthesis of ATP throughout the treatment. Several physiological processes are affected by this increase in cellular energy, including the contraction of muscles, the transmission of nerve signals, and the repair of cells.

Metabolic Regulation:

ATP synthesis can also be influenced by PEMF through the control of cellular metabolism, which is another way. Through the optimization of metabolic pathways, PEMF guarantees that cells convert nutrients into energy in an effective manner, hence contributing to the overall health and function of the cells throughout the body.

- **Improved Blood Circulation**

The influence that PEMF therapy has on blood circulation is a significant contributor to the efficacy of this treatment in facilitating healing and enhancing overall well-being.

Vasodilation and Microcirculation:

Vasodilation, or the widening of blood vessels, has been demonstrated to be induced by the electromagnetic fields produced by PEMF devices. By improving blood flow and microcirculation, this action makes sure that tissues get enough oxygen and nutrients. Increased circulation is especially important for illnesses where symptoms are exacerbated by reduced blood flow.

Blood Pressure Regulation:

Physical electromagnetic field (PEMF) therapy may be able to help regulate blood pressure, according to research. When combined with the relaxation of smooth muscle cells in blood vessels, the vasodilatory actions have the potential to result in a blood pressure profile that is more healthy and balanced.

Mental and Emotional Well-being

PEMF therapy has an impact that extends beyond the world of the physical, covering mental and emotional well-being as well because of its influence. Recognizing the interdependence of the mind and body, this holistic approach takes into consideration characteristics of stress, mood, and sleep when treating patients.

- **Stress Reduction**

Cortisol Modulation:

The effects of PEMF therapy on the stress hormone cortisol have been investigated. According to research, PEMF can regulate cortisol levels and encourage a more balanced reaction to stress. This impact helps to lessen the negative effects that prolonged stress has on the body and mind.

Neurotransmitter Regulation:

PEMF influences stress through several different mechanisms, one of which is the modification of neurotransmitters like serotonin and dopamine. These neurotransmitters play an important part in the regulation of mood, and the activity of these neurotransmitters in a balanced manner adds to an enhanced ability to withstand stress.

- **Sleep Improvement**

Circadian Rhythm Alignment:

The possibility of PEMF therapy to synchronize circadian rhythms—the innate cycles that govern sleep-wake patterns—has been investigated. PEMF has the potential to improve sleep quality and promote more restful evenings by altering melatonin synthesis and increasing relaxation.

Insomnia and Sleep Disorders:

Treatment with pulsed electromagnetic fields (PEMF) may assist people who suffer from sleep problems and insomnia. When it comes to those who are battling sleep difficulties, the relaxing effects on the nervous system and the maintenance of a healthy sleep-wake cycle can be very effective.

CHAPTER 3: DEVICES AND TECHNOLOGIES

PEMF devices are available in a variety of styles, each designed to satisfy unique requirements and tastes. Anyone thinking about incorporating PEMF therapy into their wellness routines should be aware of the broad categories of these devices.

Portable vs. Stationary Devices

Portable Devices:

Portable PEMF devices are designed for ease and adaptability. These devices are ideal for people who desire the flexibility to perform PEMF therapy at home or on the go because they are usually lightweight, rechargeable, and compact. To target specific body parts, portable devices typically take the shape of little mats or handheld applicators.

These devices' portability makes them more accessible and makes it easier for consumers to integrate PEMF therapy into their regular routines. People who value mobility and want the freedom to use PEMF wherever and whenever needed are particularly fond of them.

Stationary Devices:

On the other hand, stationary PEMF devices are larger systems made to be used in a set area, such as a clinic or residence. These gadgets could be full-body mats, mattresses, or seats that cover the entire body completely. In comparison to their portable equivalents, stationary devices frequently offer more sophisticated functions, higher intensity levels, and a wider spectrum of frequencies.

Although stationary devices are less portable, they are ideal for people who would rather have a specific area set aside for their PEMF sessions or who want more thorough and engaging therapeutic experiences. Professional PEMF treatments are also frequently administered in clinics and healthcare centers using stationary machines.

Consumer vs. Clinical Devices

Consumer Devices:

Personal usage is the intended purpose of consumer-grade PEMF devices, which enable people to manage their health and well-being from the comfort of their own homes. These gadgets have easy-to-use controls and pre-programmed settings that accommodate a range of health objectives. Consumer electronics are accessible to a diverse variety of consumers because they frequently include guidance and recommendations tailored to particular situations.

Small mats, cushions, or applicators that target particular body parts are examples of consumer gadgets. For those who are unfamiliar with PEMF therapy, they offer a gentle introduction to the modality because they are often less powerful than clinical-grade devices.

Clinical Devices:

Clinical-grade PEMF machines are more advanced and potent, and they are frequently utilized under medical professionals' guidance. These gadgets are used in medical offices, spas, and rehab clinics where skilled professionals may customize treatment to meet each patient's needs. Clinical equipment enables more precise and focused treatments by providing a wider frequency range, higher intensity settings, and sophisticated programming possibilities.

Full-body mats, specialized equipment for certain therapeutic goals, or targeted applicators are examples of clinical-grade PEMF devices. Clinical devices are appropriate for people with complex health issues or those seeking more extensive therapies since the knowledge and experience of healthcare professionals guarantee the safe and successful administration of therapy.

Popular PEMF Technologies

It is necessary to have a solid understanding of the technologies that are utilized in PEMF devices to make educated decisions on the selection of devices. Magnetic Resonance Therapy, Electrical Stimulation Therapy, and Electromagnetic Field Mat Technology are three of the most well-known types of PEMF technology.

- **Magnetic Resonance Therapy**

Principle of Magnetic Resonance:

The electromagnetic resonance theory underpins magnetic resonance therapy (MRT). It entails subjecting the body to magnetic fields that pulse and resonate with particular cells and tissues. This resonance amplifies cellular activity, stimulating multiple biological processes and facilitating ion exchange.

Applications:

MRT is adaptable and can be utilized to achieve a wide range of health objectives. The control of pain, the rebuilding of bone and tissue, and overall well-being are all prominent applications of this substance. Additionally, the resonant frequencies that are utilized in MRT are frequently set with great care to target particular tissues, which enables this technology to be adapted to a variety of therapeutic goals.

Devices:

Handheld applicators and full-body mats are only two examples of the many different types of MRT devices that are available. In the context of targeted applications, handheld devices are frequently utilized since they enable users to guide the therapy to particular regions of the body. The use of full-body mats offers a more all-encompassing experience because they administer magnetic resonance therapy to the complete body at the same time.

- **Electrical Stimulation Therapy**

Principle of Electrical Stimulation:

Electrical Stimulation Therapy, often known as EST, is where controlled electrical currents are applied to the body to stimulate the body. Nerves and muscles are stimulated by these currents, which results in the elicitation of particular physiological reactions. Electrical stimulation is utilized in the context of PEMF therapy to improve cellular function, stimulate circulation, and regulate the feeling of pain.

Applications:

The use of EST is very useful for the treatment of neurological diseases, as well as the management of pain and muscular rehabilitation. Physiological processes that occur naturally can be imitated by regulated electrical impulses, which in turn stimulate the body's natural healing systems. To provide a more all-encompassing therapeutic approach, this technology is frequently utilized in conjunction with magnetic resonance therapy treatment.

Devices:

Applicators that are handled, pads, or specialized equipment that is developed for specific uses are all examples of devices that can be used for electrical stimulation therapy. It is possible to administer targeted treatments using these devices because they can send precise electrical impulses to particular locations. Certain devices can customize settings, allowing the user to alter the intensity and frequency of electrical stimulation to meet their specific requirements.

- **Electromagnetic Field Mat Technology**

Principle of Mat Technology:

With electromagnetic field mat technology, PEMF devices are incorporated into mats or cushions that people can sit or lie on. The body is penetrated by the pulsed electromagnetic fields that these mats emit, offering a comprehensive and all-encompassing therapeutic experience. The idea is to concurrently expose every part of the body to the therapeutic benefits of PEMF.

Applications:

The flexible mat technology provides advantages for better sleep, stress relief, and general well-being. Users can easily include

PEMF therapy into their everyday routines by simply relaxing on the mat while it is being administered. Mat technology is also applied to larger cellular function enhancement and pain control.

Devices:

Magnetic Field Mats are available in a range of shapes and sizes. While some are smaller mats intended for specialized uses, others are full-body mats that people can lie on. These mats frequently have pre-programmed settings and varying intensities, enabling users to customize their therapy sessions to meet their health objectives.

Considerations for Choosing a PEMF Device

When thinking about purchasing a PEMF device, there are a few things that should be taken into consideration:

1. Health Goals:

Determine your unique health objectives and the ailments you hope PEMF therapy may help with. It's important to match the technology and gadget you choose with your health goals, as some may be better suited for specific aims.

2. Intensity and Frequency Range:

Take into consideration the various intensity levels and frequency ranges that the instrument provides. It is crucial to select a device that is to your unique requirements, as the best settings may change depending on the health situation.

3. Portability and Convenience:

Choose between having a device that is stationary for a more immersive experience or a gadget that is portable for more flexibility. While fixed devices can be used at home, portable devices are required for individuals who wish to undergo PEMF therapy while they are on the go.

4. User-Friendly Controls:

Make sure the equipment has controls that are easy to use and clear directions. Consumer electronics should be simple to use, but healthcare equipment could have more sophisticated features that need expert assistance.

5. Safety Features:

Verify that safety elements including temperature control, automated shut-off systems, and adherence to safety regulations are present. When choosing a PEMF device, safety should always come first, particularly for personal use.

6. Professional Guidance:

Seek advice from medical specialists or PEMF therapy practitioners if you have complicated medical conditions or unique health concerns. They can guarantee the technology is used safely and effectively and offer tailored recommendations.

CHAPTER 4: CHOOSING THE RIGHT PEMF DEVICE

An essential step in maximizing the benefits of this therapy modality is making sure that the Pulsed Electromagnetic Field (PEMF) device that you use is appropriately calibrated. Individuals are required to take into consideration their particular health objectives, individual health conditions, and technical specifications when selecting a device from the vast selection of options that are currently available, which range from portable consumer options to clinical-grade equipment. The purpose of this in-depth tutorial is to examine the most important aspects to take into consideration when selecting a PEMF device for personal use.

Considerations for Personal Use

- ***Specific Health Goals***

Setting clear health objectives is the most important factor to take into account when selecting a PEMF device. PEMF therapy is adaptable and can be used to treat many different types of health issues. For some goals, other gadgets and technologies might be more appropriate. The following are typical health objectives and the factors to be taken into account for each:

Pain Management:

Consider equipment that offers focused application options, like handheld applicators or pads, if pain control is the main objective. To customize the therapy to the patient's level of pain, look for devices with adjustable intensity levels and frequencies that are known to have analgesic benefits.

Bone and Tissue Regeneration:

Devices with a spectrum of frequencies that promote cellular proliferation and differentiation are helpful for those who are focused on bone and tissue regeneration. Localized applicators or full-body mats may be appropriate for targeting particular trouble spots.

Stress Reduction and Relaxation:

Devices with lower frequencies linked to relaxing effects may be helpful for people looking to reduce stress and unwind. One option to consider is the use of equipment with pre-programmed relaxation settings or magnetic field mats.

Enhanced Cellular Function:

It is recommended to use devices that offer a variety of frequencies and intensity levels to improve the overall operation of the cell. To give extensive covering for a holistic approach to cellular wellbeing, full-body mats or mats with a variety of applicators can be utilized.

Improved Sleep:

It may be good for people who are having trouble sleeping to choose a gadget that has features that match the circadian cycle and frequencies that are calming. Electromagnetic field mats designed to improve sleep quality might be helpful in this situation.

▪ Individual Health Conditions

Every person's unique health circumstances are a crucial factor in deciding which PEMF device is the most appropriate for them. Some things to take into account based on typical health issues are as follows:

Arthritis or Joint Pain:

People with arthritis or joint pain may find relief from their discomfort with devices that include frequencies known for their anti-inflammatory qualities. Providing focused relief to damaged joints can be accomplished with the help of portable devices such as handheld applicators or tiny mats.

Sports Injuries:

Individuals who are recuperating from sports injuries may find that devices that provide a combination of magnetic resonance therapy and electrical stimulation therapy are beneficial to their recovery. If you want to personalize the therapy to different stages of recovery, you might think about using portable devices that have settings that can be customized.

Chronic Conditions:

The use of clinical-grade devices, which are administered under the supervision of medical specialists, may be beneficial to individuals who suffer from chronic diseases. It is common for these devices to offer higher intensity levels and more complex programming options that are ideal for long-term control.

Osteoporosis:

Devices that strengthen bone density and promote bone regeneration are necessary for people who suffer from osteoporosis. Individuals who suffer from this illness may benefit from the broad covering that can be provided by full-body mats that provide a variety of frequencies.

Stress-Related Conditions:

If you are coping with conditions that are related to stress, it is essential to select a device that has frequencies that are known for their ability to reduce tension. When it comes to stress management on the go, portable equipment that allows for flexibility in use, such as handheld applicators, may be effective.

Evaluating Technical Specifications

The evaluation of the technical characteristics of PEMF devices becomes extremely important after health goals and other individual factors have been taken into consideration. By having a thorough understanding of the technical aspects, one can verify that the equipment selected is following the outcomes that are wanted, as well as being safe and effective for personal usage.

- **Frequency Ranges**

When it comes to PEMF therapy, frequency is an essential component since different frequencies evoke varied physiological reactions from the body. When thinking about frequency ranges, take into consideration the following aspects:

Wide Range of Frequencies:

Pick out a device that provides access to a diverse variety of frequencies. The adaptability of this product makes it possible to tailor it to fit particular health objectives. The ability to address a wide variety of health conditions is made possible by the availability of devices that have frequencies that range from low (for relaxation) to high (for cellular stimulation).

Targeted Frequencies:

It is important to look for medical devices that include particular frequencies that are known for their therapeutic effects for treating specific health disorders. As a means of guiding the choosing process, research on the best frequencies for specific health goals can be helpful.

Pulsed or Continuous Waveforms:

Find out whether the gadget produces continuous waves or pulsed waveforms. In the field of PEMF therapy, pulsed waveforms, which are characterized by occasional bursts of energy, are frequently used. Certain gadgets may provide the capability to switch between pulsed and continuous modes according to the preferences of the user of the device.

- **Intensity Levels**

The strength of the magnetic field that is produced by the device can be determined by its intensity, which can be measured in either Gauss or Tesla. When thinking about intensity levels, take into consideration the following aspects:

Adjustable Intensity:

Select a gadget that offers several intensity settings. Users can begin with lesser intensities and progressively increase them as needed thanks to this functionality. It's crucial to have adjustable intensity if you're new to PEMF therapy or have sensitivity issues.

High Intensity for Specific Conditions:

In cases of chronic pain or musculoskeletal disorders, increased intensity levels could be advantageous. Higher intensities are frequently offered by clinical-grade equipment, making them appropriate for patients who need more powerful treatment.

Safety Measures:

Look for intensity-related safety features like automated shut-off mechanisms or alerts for excessive intensity. When employing PEMF devices, safety should always come first, and the intensity levels should only be utilized sparingly.

- **Duration of Sessions**

The length of PEMF therapy sessions can affect the treatment's overall efficacy. Examine the following factors that affect how long a session lasts:

Flexible Session Durations:

Choose a gadget that gives you the ability to decide how long your sessions will last. While shorter sessions could be appropriate for general wellness, longer sessions might be more beneficial for some diseases. Convenience can be achieved with the use of devices consisting of programmable timers or pre-set session durations.

Guidelines for Specific Conditions:

To determine the ideal duration of sessions for specific health issues, it is recommended that you consult the guidelines or suggestions. Certain devices may come with documents or instructions that provide information regarding the recommended length for addressing specific health concerns.

Consistency in Usage:

Consistently using the PEMF device is frequently essential to getting the benefits that are intended. To ensure that implementing PEMF therapy into your routine is not only possible but also fun, it is important to choose a device that is compatible with your living situation and

personal preferences.

CHAPTER 5: USING PEMF THERAPY SAFELY

PEMF therapy, which stands for pulsed electromagnetic field, is widely regarded as a non-invasive and safe treatment option. It is vital, however, to use PEMF devices responsibly to assure both safety and effectiveness, just as it is with any other therapeutic method. In order to assist persons in securely using PEMF therapy, this thorough guide covers common issues, discusses session protocols, and discusses a variety of precautions and contraindications.

Precautions and Contraindications

- **Pregnancy and Breastfeeding**

Pregnancy:

It is typically recommended that pregnant individuals refrain from using PEMF devices, particularly during the first trimester of their pregnancy. This is even though there is a limited amount of data on the effects of PEMF therapy during pregnancy. The possibility that electromagnetic fields could affect embryos that are still developing is a cause for concern, and it is recommended that women exercise caution to protect both themselves and their unborn children.

Breastfeeding:

Likewise, scant information exists regarding PEMF therapy's safety during lactation. Breastfeeding mothers should exercise caution when using PEMF therapy and should speak with a healthcare provider first. In this case, the possible effect on the growing neurological system of the baby is taken into account.

- **Implantable Devices**

Pacemakers and Implantable Cardioverter Defibrillators (ICDs):

When utilizing PEMF devices, people with pacemakers or ICDs should use caution because electromagnetic fields can interfere with the functionality of these implanted devices. To ascertain whether utilizing PEMF therapy in conjunction with such implants is safe, it is imperative to speak with a medical professional and the device maker.

Other Implants:

It is also important for those who have other kinds of implants, such as brain stimulators or cochlear implants, to take caution. Before beginning to use PEMF therapy, it is important to seek the counsel of a specialist because the influence of electromagnetic fields on the operation of these devices is something that should be taken into consideration.

- **Neurological Conditions**

Seizure Disorders:

When utilizing PEMF therapy, anyone with a history of seizures or epilepsy should exercise caution. Even if there is conflicting information on the connection between PEMF therapy and seizures, it is still advised to speak with a healthcare provider before beginning PEMF sessions, particularly when the intensity is higher.

Migraines:

PEMF therapy may cause or worsen headaches in certain people, therefore those who are prone to migraines or severe headaches should use it with caution. It is advised to begin with lower intensities and shorter durations while keeping an eye out for any negative effects.

Guidelines for Session Protocols

- **Frequency and Duration Recommendations**

General Guidelines:

Depending on the objectives and circumstances of each patient, there are differences in the ideal frequency and length of PEMF treatments. Generally speaking, it's best to begin with shorter sessions (10–20 minutes), and then progressively extend them. For chronic diseases, longer sessions might be an option, but the choice should be based on each patient's tolerance and response.

Frequency Selection:

To achieve the intended therapeutic benefits, choosing the right frequencies is essential.

Making use of existing material or speaking with medical experts might help with frequency selection based on particular health objectives. Lower frequencies linked to relaxation may be appropriate for overall health, whereas higher frequencies may be more focused on cellular stimulation.

- **Monitoring and Adjusting Intensity**

Adjustable Intensity:

Select a PEMF device that allows you to easily modify the intensity levels. Users can begin with lesser intensities thanks to this function, which is especially helpful for those who are new to PEMF therapy or who are struggling with sensitivity difficulties. A secure and comfortable experience can be ensured by gradually raising the intensity of the workout as the body adjusts to it.

Individual Sensitivity:

PEMF therapy susceptibility varies from person to person. While some people could find it uncomfortable at lesser intensities, others might be able to handle higher levels effectively. A safe and enjoyable experience depends on paying attention to the body's reaction and modifying the intensity appropriately.

Monitoring for Adverse Effects:

People should keep an eye out for any negative side effects, such as headaches, nausea, or dizziness, both during and after PEMF sessions. If these symptoms happen, it can mean that the length or intensity has to be changed. If severe or long-lasting side effects are noticed, it is best to speak with a healthcare provider.

Addressing Common Concerns and Misconceptions

1. PEMF Therapy and Cancer:

Concern: Some people are concerned that PEMF treatment could encourage the growth of cancer cells.

Evidence: There is conflicting evidence about the connection between PEMF therapy and cancer. While some studies indicate no discernible effect, others point to possible anti-cancer effects. For those with a history of cancer, consulting an oncologist is advised.

2. PEMF Therapy and EMF Exposure:

Concern: People could be concerned about the possible health hazards linked to electromagnetic field exposure (EMFs).

Mitigation: Low-frequency electromagnetic fields (EMFs) are emitted by PEMF devices, as opposed to higher-frequency EMFs from electronic gadgets. To reduce worries about excessive EMF exposure, select devices with low-intensity settings, use them at a safe distance, and schedule pauses in between sessions.

3. PEMF Therapy and Medications:

Concern: Users can worry if PEMF therapy and drugs interact.

Guidance: Even while PEMF therapy is usually regarded as safe, it is still essential to speak with a healthcare provider, particularly if you are on medication. Certain drugs may interfere with PEMF therapy, and a medical professional can offer tailored advice depending on a patient's specific health issues.

4. PEMF Therapy and Acute Injuries:

Concern: People might wonder if PEMF treatment is appropriate for recent injuries.

Application: For acute injuries, PEMF therapy can help reduce inflammation and accelerate healing. But it's important to begin with shorter durations and lower intensities and work your way up to a higher level as the injury recovers. Expert advice could be helpful in situations involving recent injuries.

5. PEMF Therapy and Chronic Conditions:

Concern: Users can doubt PEMF therapy's effectiveness in treating long-term illnesses.

Consideration: Pain, arthritis, and neurological diseases are just a few of the chronic ailments that PEMF therapy has shown promise in treating. The efficacy of PEMF therapy for long-term health issues is dependent on user consistency, adherence to suggested regimens, and expert advice.

CHAPTER 6: CASE STUDIES AND SUCCESS STORIES

Pulsed electromagnetic field therapy, also known as PEMF therapy, has gained a lot of attention because it has the potential to reduce pain, aid in rehabilitation, and improve general well-being. As we explore deeper into real-life experiences and expert testimonials, we uncover the different uses of PEMF therapy as well as the excellent effects that have been recorded by individuals from a wide range of backgrounds.

Real-Life Experiences with PEMF Therapy

- Pain Management

Case Study 1: Chronic Back Pain Relief

Sarah, a 45-year-old employee in an office, has been enduring persistent lower back discomfort for several years. The alleviation offered by conventional therapy was just momentary. She decided to add a portable PEMF device to her regimen after becoming intrigued by the possibility of this therapy. Following many weeks of consistent use, Sarah saw a notable alleviation of her back pain. Her general range of motion and flexibility were enhanced by the therapy in addition to relieving her discomfort.

Case Study 2: Arthritic Joint Pain

John, a sixty-year-old retiree, was told he had osteoarthritis, which was causing his knees to hurt and become stiff. He began using a PEMF mat at home as a substitute for painkillers. John saw observable changes over the next few months. His knees became less tight, and he was able to do things he had not done before. The possibility of PEMF therapy as a non-invasive treatment option for arthritic joint pain is demonstrated by John's case.

- **Sports Recovery**

Case Study 3: Faster Healing After an Injury

A professional athlete named Mark hurt his hamstrings in training. He added PEMF therapy to his rehabilitation regimen in an attempt to speed up his recuperation. Mark saw a quicker healing process by combining full-body mat sessions with focused PEMF applications. The treatment was vital in promoting muscle regeneration in addition to lowering discomfort and inflammation. Mark credited PEMF therapy for his quicker recovery and went back to training earlier than anticipated.

Case Study 4: Enhanced Endurance and Performance

Emily, an amateur marathon runner, struggled with exhaustion and a protracted recovery period following extended races. She started utilizing a handheld PEMF device after exercise because she was intrigued by the possible advantages of PEMF therapy on sports performance. Emily felt less discomfort in her muscles and increased endurance. Her ability to train more regularly as a result of the therapy helped her achieve better overall performance and race times.

- **Chronic Health Conditions**

Case Study 5: Improved Quality of Life with Fibromyalgia

After receiving a fibromyalgia diagnosis, Alexandra experienced weariness, irregular sleep patterns, and persistent discomfort. There was little alleviation from traditional therapy. She attempted PEMF therapy with a full-body mat, despite her skepticism. As time went on, Alexandra's symptoms significantly improved. She experienced less pain and more peaceful sleep. Consistent PEMF therapy use helped Alexandra's quality of life to improve and became an essential part of her self-care regimen.

Case Study 6: Managing Neuropathic Pain in Diabetes

James, a patient with diabetes, experienced neuropathic pain in his feet, which affected his day-to-day activities. In search of alternatives to painkillers, he investigated PEMF treatment. James was able to get relief from neuropathic pain in his feet by using localized PEMF applications. His general sense of wellbeing was enhanced by the therapy in addition to lessening the degree of his discomfort. James's story demonstrates how PEMF therapy may be used to treat neuropathic pain brought on by long-term illnesses.

Professional Testimonials

- **Healthcare Practitioners**

Testimonial 1: Integrating PEMF Therapy in Pain Management

PEMF therapy was incorporated into Dr. Patel's practice as a pain management specialist to give patients with chronic pain more options. Having seen successful results in multiple instances, he revealed, "PEMF therapy is now a useful addition to our pain management strategy. For patients who might not tolerate or react well to conventional therapies, it provides a non-invasive option. Some of our patients have seen improvements in their general quality of life, greater mobility, and pain scores."

Testimonial 2: Supporting Rehabilitation in Physical Therapy

Physical therapist Rebecca added PEMF treatment to her patients' rehabilitation regimens as they healed from wounds. She pointed out, "We have found PEMF therapy to be an invaluable resource in our physical therapy practice. It expedites the healing process and enhances conventional therapies. PEMF therapy has been shown to shorten recovery durations, increase range of motion, and improve muscular function in patients undergoing rehabilitation."

- **Athletes and Celebrities**

Testimonial 3: Professional Athlete's Endorsement

A well-known professional athlete with a track record of reaching optimal performance levels discussed the benefits of PEMF therapy for recuperation. "In the realm of professional athletics, recuperation is an essential component of success. For years, I have included PEMF therapy into my routine, and it has changed everything. It enables me to recuperate more quickly from demanding training sessions and contests, enabling me to continuously perform at my best."

Testimonial 4: Celebrity Wellness Journey with PEMF

A well-known celebrity who prioritizes holistic health gave details about their PEMF therapy experience. "Being in the spotlight can be demanding, so preserving general wellbeing must come first. I've experimented with several health techniques, but PEMF treatment has been a regular part of my regimen. It contributes to a balanced and healthful lifestyle by enhancing my mental and physical well-being."

CHAPTER 7: FUTURE TRENDS AND DEVELOPMENTS

Even though Pulsed Electromagnetic Field (PEMF) therapy can alter cellular function and aid healing, it is still a subject of investigation and innovation. As we look to the future, we can see that the current landscape of PEMF therapy is being shaped by several fascinating trends and advancements. This all-encompassing investigation digs into the rising frontiers of this dynamic area, covering topics such as the integration of PEMF therapy with traditional medicine as well as continuing research and clinical trials.

Ongoing Research and Clinical Trials

- **Emerging Applications**

Neurological Disorders:

The use of PEMF therapy to treat neurological problems is being investigated in more and more neurology-related research. Studies on the effects of PEMF on ailments such as traumatic brain injuries, Parkinson's disease, and Alzheimer's disease are still ongoing. According to preliminary research, PEMF therapy may affect neural activity and have neuroprotective benefits.

Autoimmune Diseases:

PEMF therapy is showing promise in the treatment of autoimmune illnesses by potentially modifying the immune response.

The effects of PEMF on diseases like multiple sclerosis, lupus, and rheumatoid arthritis are being investigated in preliminary research. The objective is to comprehend the potential role that PEMF therapy may play in immune control and the relief of autoimmune disease symptoms.

Metabolic Disorders:

There is growing interest in the application of PEMF therapy to metabolic diseases like obesity and diabetes. The purpose of the study is to look into how PEMF affects adipose tissue function, insulin sensitivity, and cellular metabolism. These investigations could shed light on how PEMF promotes metabolic health and treats illnesses associated with energy balance imbalance.

- Advancements in Technology

Personalized PEMF Protocols:

Personalized PEMF procedures are becoming possible thanks to technological advancements. Future PEMF devices might allow customization based on a person's health profile as researchers learn more about how different frequencies and intensities affect individual responses. This customized strategy seeks to maximize therapeutic results and raise PEMF therapy's general efficacy.

Integration of Wearable Technology:

An emerging trend is the integration of PEMF technology with wearable devices. Researchers are investigating the possibility of integrating tiny PEMF devices into wearables like patches or smartwatches. Because of this integration, people may easily implement PEMF therapy into their regular routines and receive on-the-go wellness support.

Advancements in Delivery Systems:

PEMF therapy is becoming more widely accessible thanks to advancements in delivery technologies. Users' options are being expanded by new device designs such as small applicators, flexible mats, and garment-integrated technologies. With the help of these developments, PEMF therapy should become easier to utilize, enabling patients to easily cover their entire body or target particular locations.

Integration with Conventional Medicine

- **Collaborative Approaches**

Complementary Therapy in Pain Management:

A growing number of people are becoming interested in collaborative methods that combine PEMF therapy with traditional pain management techniques. Clinics that treat pain and provide rehabilitation are investigating the potential benefits of combining PEMF therapy with other therapies like physiotherapy, acupuncture, or medicine. The overall goals of this integrative strategy are to improve patient outcomes and offer complete pain relief.

Adjunct to Orthopedic Interventions:

PEMF therapy is being explored as a surgical and non-surgical intervention adjunct in orthopedics. Research is looking into the use of PEMF therapy in pre and post-operative care to improve results for procedures including spinal surgery and joint replacements by reducing inflammation and promoting healing. PEMF therapy has been shown by orthopedic doctors to help rehabilitation and speed up recovery.

Incorporation into Mental Health Practices:

Mental health practitioners are exploring the incorporation of PEMF therapy into the management of stress, anxiety, and mood disorders. Collaborative efforts between mental health professionals and PEMF practitioners aim to develop evidence-based protocols for integrating PEMF therapy into psychotherapy and wellness programs. Preliminary studies suggest that PEMF therapy may have a positive impact on mental well-being by influencing neurotransmitter levels and neuroplasticity.

CONCLUSION

PEMF therapy emerges not only as a therapeutic modality but also as a paradigm that coincides with the holistic approach to health and wellness. In conclusion, PEMF therapy is considered to be a paradigm. The journey through its foundations, health benefits, device selection, safety protocols, real-life experiences, and future trends highlights the intricate tapestry that PEMF therapy weaves within the larger landscape of natural and non-invasive health interventions. PEMF therapy is a form of electromagnetic field (EMF) therapy.

For individuals to successfully navigate this landscape, it is essential to approach PEMF therapy with a well-informed viewpoint, acknowledging both its promise and its limitations. Safety should continue to be the most important factor to take into account, and working together with medical professionals can provide individualized guidance that is customized to the specific requirements of each individual's health.

Both practitioners and users are encouraged to keep up with the latest developments in PEMF therapy and to contribute to the overall understanding of its mechanisms and applications. This is because the nature of PEMF therapy is such that it is constantly evolving, which encourages continuous exploration and research. In the course of this ongoing journey, the combination of scientific investigation, technological advancement, and personal experiences serves as the basis for a future in which PEMF therapy may play an increasingly important role in promoting well-being across a wide range of populations.

In conclusion, as we come to the end of this investigation, the door is still wide open for additional discoveries, improvements, and a more in-depth comprehension of the complex ways in which PEMF therapy may contribute to the quest for a life that is both healthier and more lively.